內 力 智 安

gwynneth green

**Wasteland Press**
Shelbyville, KY USA
www.wastelandpress.net

*Inner Strength, Widsom, Tranquility:*
*A Meditation & Yoga Companion*
by Gwynneth Green

Copyright © 2009 Gwynneth Green
ALL RIGHTS RESERVED

First Printing—July 2009
ISBN: 978-1-60047-331-9



Printed in the U.S.A.

*"The pieces in this companion are a transformational reflective tool. Each verse can be read aloud during a group practice as I do during my Zen teachings, or in solitude. The author inspires us during these times of uncertainty in the world with soulful expressions and takes us on a journey to inner strength and tranquility. Gwynneth Green's words are sensitive and evocative and a must read for anyone interested in enhanced spirituality and meditation."*

Bankei Nora Dellacroce, Ph.D.
Usui  Reiki Mastership
Faculty Member, Zen Society

*"Gwynneth Green's extraordinary gift of profound, free-flowing expression is deeply connected to her family legacy. Carrying on her grandfather Bud's tradition of uniquely original lyrical gifting, Gwynneth has blazed her own passionate trail during the past few decades. Breathing deeply and rhythmically, Gwynneth's evocative observations warm the heart, feed the soul, and gently rattle the conscious mind."*

Robert Parish
Author
Award-winning Independent Filmmaker

*"Gwynneth Green lends a perfect voice to yoga.  Her concise and rhythmic style of writing sets an intention to the practice in the same manner as breath to the movement of asana. Gwynneth's poetry read aloud at the beginning of savasana helps my students deepen their practice by providing a stillpoint to calm the body/mind."*

Cara McGray RYT

meditative mood

the meditative mood
a breath to refresh
a breath to cleanse
exhale....
hurt
ache
& pain
reclaim
existence
finding creation
your own universe

heave thoughts
that tug your mind
immerse self
to self inside

build a room
suiting needs
windows
that allow a breeze
a scent recognized
realizing
it's your own
this place
in self
is home
protected
by
goodness & grace
blessed
by
virtue............. embrace
calm
flooding every cell
weights lift
mind drifts
let go
let go

a breath to refresh
a breath to cleanse
reclaim
existence
your own universe

# table of contents

内力

inner strength

your voice

let not a negative thought near
doing damage
to 1's soul
conquer
take control
for in a silent moment
when breath
can't be heard
heart so still
will
stronger than before
adoration found
in dreams of day
placed neatly
surrounding
drowning
anxiety
which……..way
when you think your lost
the pool is clear
the reflection
mere….ly
stares back
lacking
the ability to speak………..??
peer deeper
for the eyes are yours
as is the voice
if only heard
no sound to mute
for  thunder blares within
listen
listen
a deaf ear hears the same
the voice
calls out your name
the voice
leads every direction
and remains
your voice………..your heart
your soul

there are no keys
for there
are no doors
no boundaries
limits
restrictions
anymore

Green, <u>unsung songs,</u> p.2

be still


forgot how to feel
reality is real
close
to your soul
a heart…….. not just a pump
it lumps
sorrow & pain
happiness remains
choose today
not tomorrow or the next
lay a path
from smiles within
lay a path


peace
is not behind a door
stored serenity
to obtain
let
your mind be still
cast
adversarial thoughts
a will……ingness
to surrender
peace
calm
ease
be still

passage from<br>a wish

skip
no run
in the direction
of
sunny days
ocean's sprays
that
trickle
on the pores
of dressless skin
linger
in the water's light
that caresses
ankles hips and more

Green, <u>unsung songs,</u> p.36

re-capture


re-captured life
in a dew drop
on a leaf
the web of friends
tied by a strand
smiles…….not taken for granted
miles
a distant covered quickly
by thought
anxieties collected…….. scattered
then tossed
who are we
to question why
accepting each others
cries
belong to the whole
mine
are yours
to coddle
hold……. each
tear a binding thread
a joyful dance
blends
ages yet shared
&
re-captured times
left
left
less………..defined

relax


relax your mind
let go of the weight of your limbs
the energy
from your soul
flows through your skin
spread you fingers
let lingering troubles
escape
no longer trapped with in
finding a calm place
solitude's not emptiness
rather an embrace
finding your other self
in your own retreat
sounds heard
are meaningless
they lack a track or trace
no thoughts to bother
they're easily replaced
the breath is silent
serene
sedate
nothing wakes this world
take with it
tranquility
shed all that disturbs
relax
relax
a moment more
relax
relax
your energy restored

passage from
imprint

15

my imprints left
upon the beach
no longer
attached to my feet
winds shift
and scatter sands
solid………. my am

soul's intact
matters not where i roam
for in all senses
my heart is home

Green, <u>unsung songs II,</u> p.

*passage from*
ask


fall
not away
not so far
hitting bottom
hurts…….less
when focusing
the best
is yet to come

Green, <u>unsung songs II,</u> p.

worry


worry
where does it send you
into turmoil
depression
agitating your soul
spreading
it out
to others
unknown
capturing
trapping
you into despair
where does it send you
nowhere............
that i shall be
what bothers
see it
set it free
who is in control
a worry bug
that takes & doles
out pain
as if drugged
no
no
no
be
the master
of your soul
ascertain
your goal

haiku #4



unconditional
 care
      sincerity
            sharing
love's ingredients

智

wisdom

you smiled


did you laugh
with life today
take in stride
try not to hide
let sorrow find
a different venue
finding a tune
that lifts
drifts
from note to note
denoting
a change
in
the pattern
of syncopated rain
see
you smiled
at me
not even questioning why
it's the freedom
you dared
to share
in wild abandonment
forgetting
what clogged your mind
you smiled
once more
for
letting down the wall
anger has no place
this space
is graced
with affection
oh
you smiled
once more

enter
the space
waken
no limitations
only lacking imagination

Green, <u>unsung songs,</u> p.23

a token


forgot what
was asked
was it
before
or
after
the fact
yesterday
today
or
tomorrow's
news
badly taken
badly used
nothing is
a waste
of emotion
for a token
is always left
regardless
of the day
of the way
a token
for
remembering
why
the sky is always blue
the sun
remembers too
shine
when you think
your cold


look
don't stare
in the mirror
a reflection
the resurrection
of thee

reality sings

reality sings a different song
for you than for me
you view the ocean turbulent
i feel it's breeze
anger
doesn't dissipate
because the sky turned blue
a different hue
is my view though we disagree
weeping never works
doesn't change 1's mind
tears of madness
tears of sadness
and those of joy
all combine
laughter can't be tamed
not to shine or glow
have you listened
heard a word
oh
mine don't count
just yours
reality sings to me with glee
no negativities break the calm
reality is
differences
should be heard
understanding
is really not demanding
if care is a concern

*passage from*
mind set


solitude
is not the escape
search
find
the place
where peace & action
combine
letting
souls entwine
to 1

Green, <u>unsung songs II,</u> p.

sunbeams

the sun rose today
with a silent demeanor
left it's beams behind
the moon asked why
the sun replied
why not ………. i'm tired today
the moon stated
you've left the universe
dark
it is your job
to light  the way
i can not reflect
unless
you share your strength
with me
the sun
pondered a moment or 2
looking around
caught the view
of dark – dank & dismal
no laughter heard
bursting of energy
unveiling her light
shook of darkness
to the moon's delight
a ray spilled here
and another there
laughter once more
filled the air
oh
it is not only the sun
it's in your heart
when
tied & closed
feeling cold and alone
the moon is never a distance away
the moon's the friend
that always stays
reminding 1
keep your heart a glow
your beams will follow
spreading
love & laughter
to all you know

turn the page


is it shelter you seek
from what
the sorrow you keep
kept alive
from
something derived
hid …….hiding inside
refuge from years
of  wrath
an attack
that never took place
it is
your turn
to turn the page
engage
in letting go
you need not me


go
go to the place
that erases anger
displaces ire
chasing the cycle of pain
embrace
this moment
imbed the peace
weave a thread
of serene
from your limbs
settling in your head


turn the page
turn the page
engulfed
engage
in
your temperate soul

reflections refract
   attracting revelations
      enlightening we

# haiku #3

capability
inward investigation
potentials exposed

joy is for the taking

everyone needs
an answer
though the question
may vary
from day to day
results aren't a given
success is within
don't measure
more to less
for less is more
when weights are gone
the forlorn aren't forgotten
merely heaped in a pile
looking for someone
answering their fantasy
yet it's dancing in front of their eyes
the dark side of the moon
doesn't have to be lightless
the stars still twinkle
sending flicks of laughter
into the night
fright
has no claim
have you forgotten
how to smile
nothing's solved
if you dissolve
yourself in wine
what is the outcome
if you run
leaving fun
behind
sorrow
swallows the soul
leaving 1 cold
feel…………..the warmth of the sun
squeal in………..side splitting wit
admitting
joy is for the taking

安

tranquility

self


close eyes
linger
in an exhaled breath
counting
the seconds
till 1 is refreshed
the air upon pores
tickling the tiniest follicle
a mind
seemingly still
not casting off will
wallowing in the waves
of absolute calm
a moment
shared with.......self
no one else


entity
the place 1 dwells
the space
perceived
not encased or shelled
if dreams
are not reality
ambition looses


disillusionment
won't win
enlightenment
claim
seize
conquer ...............lunacy
replacing
the space
with tranquility
a moment
shared with.......self
no one else

*passage from*
wet sand


the sea
brushes me
asking nothing
giving all
clearing
mis……..
givings
understandings
stakes

gull's laughter
embrace the day
a melodic tune
to some
one
who has reach peace
under the heated sun


Green, <u>unsung songs II,</u> p.

lay still


lay still
lay still
let the calm
around
encapsulate
finding solitude
while minds
dance in delight
lay still
lay still
rose petals
cover the carpet
that leads
to the door
of fear
waken
for it does not exist
lilacs' scent
the room is filled
no place
for despair to roam
thy home
is clear
lay still
lay still
darkness seeks
to take control
the light
is one's hold
lay still
one's will
one's desire
one's passion
one's fire
united
never tires


lay still
lay still

*passage from*
smiles last longer


tears
happily
evaporate
away
no
dust
shall
settle
upon
the
waves
sweet
songs
sing
in
the
soul
bringing
hearts
warmth
from
the
cold


Green, <u>unsung songs,</u> p.8

soul's comfort



time
can't let it fly by
nor
stand………… still
each moment
lived
captured
remembered…………..
till
our hearts & minds
are filled
memories
can not be replaced
erased by future
misgivings .. undertakings
no mistaking
mine
& yours
are alike
though different
in appearance
hold
tight
to yours
and
i to mine
they may or not intertwine
a
soul's comfort
divine

i pass you the pipe
no drugs does it bare
take  a draw
inhale
the air
of universal breath

clearing the head
of unwanted clutter
leaving space
new discover....ies
fill your cup
with wishes and wants
abundance grows
with each flow
inhale
inhale
inhale
universal air

lay
with me
by water's edge
watching
the waves
lap the shore
counting
the tears
that did not fall
catching
the rays
that caress the souls

let laughter
tickle your heart
as it beats in time
with mine
spill
the words
that need the air
untying fear
the path
unmistakably clear

Green, <u>unsung songs,</u> p.34

bask in the sun


some die
some hide
others bask in the sun
never wondering
what will or won't become
taking stride
that the ride
is easy
sanity
the sanctuary


recognized or not


berserk
cracked
deranged
disturbed
feelings felt
described
by others
insanely jealous
of a mind's freedom
running rampedly wild
safe
within boundaries unseen
that slightly whacked smile
testing laughter's walls


while
others
bask in the sun

*passage from*
desire rages


step out
of the dark
into
the light
fight
fight
the urge
of discourage……..ment
waves
of laughter
spill upon
the shore
adorned
by shells
the sea
has born

Green, <u>unsung songs,</u> p.20

haiku #1



tranquil seas embrace
        societies distress quelled
oceans enchantment

quiet night


quiet night....soft thoughts.......sleep well.........no dreams

within the soft cocoon
we weave
a place of rest
protected
by calm
allow rest
to swallow
allow peace
to follow
with in
that dark night
a light always burns
pointing
directing
guiding
to ease the yearn
of loneliness
of distress
of emptiness
those are shallow
and need only to be
swept in a corner
taken with the breeze
wade into
sleep............ with no dreams
close eyes
feel no strain
warmth engulfing
relieving pain
hurt & bother
no longer persist
focus on colors
that assist in repair
focus on feelings
of love & care


quiet night....soft thoughts.......sleep well.........no dreams

strength lies
in a crying child's smile
wisdom walks
a path that's cleared
as 1 dozes
tranquility flows
through the veins
of our years


for
all those dear
to my heart
or yours

# g w y n n e t h   g r e e n

---

unsung songs
unsung songs II

www.buddinggreen.com

design work by: Monika Jakober Designs
www.monikajakoberdesigns.com

Breinigsville, PA USA
15 February 2010
232515BV00001B/2/P